Skin Care

The Ultimate Guide to Nourishing Your Skin Naturally

Table of Contents

Chapter 10

The skin care recommendations for different ages, seasons, and occasions.

Chapter 11

Skin Care secrets of celebrities and experts

Introduction

Your skin is not only a visible aspect that you can beautify or ignore. It is a vital organ that influences your health, wellness, and self-confidence. Your skin displays your inner condition and emotions, and it safeguards you from harmful elements, such as sun, pollution, bacteria, and allergens. That is why caring for your skin properly is important for your well-being.

This means that skin care is not a superficial or extravagant activity. It is a way of taking care of yourself, your health, and your happiness. Your skin is the biggest organ of your body, and it mirrors your inner state of being. It also acts as a barrier from external factors, such as sun, pollution, bacteria, and allergens. Therefore, looking after your skin well is essential for your overall well-being.

But how do you know what is the best skin care routine for you? How do you choose the right products, ingredients, and techniques for your skin type, concerns, and goals? How do you balance your skin care needs with your lifestyle, budget, and preferences? How do you avoid common skin care mistakes and myths that can harm your skin and waste your money?

This means that finding the best skin care routine for you is not a simple or easy task. It requires some research, experimentation, and evaluation. You need to know your skin type, concerns, and goals, and choose the products, ingredients, and techniques that suit them. You also need to consider your lifestyle, budget, and preferences, and find a balance between your skin care needs and your personal circumstances. You also need to be aware of the common skin care mistakes and myths that can damage your skin and waste your money.

That is what this book is all about. Skin Care and You is a comprehensive guide that will help you understand your skin better, and provide you with practical and effective solutions for your skin care challenges. Whether you want to prevent or treat acne, wrinkles, dryness, sensitivity, or any other skin issue, this book will show you how to achieve healthy, radiant, and beautiful skin.

This means that this book is your ultimate resource for skin care. Skin Care and You is a complete guide that will help you learn more about your skin, and offer you realistic and effective solutions for your skin care problems. Whether you want to prevent or treat acne, wrinkles, dryness, sensitivity, or any other skin issue, this book will teach you how to achieve healthy, radiant, and beautiful skin.

Chapter 1

The basics of skin anatomy, physiology, and function

The basics of skin anatomy, physiology, and function is a topic that explains the structure, function, and behavior of your skin, which is the largest organ of your body. It covers the following aspects:

The layers of your skin and their roles: Your skin has three main layers: the epidermis, the dermis, and the hypodermis. The epidermis is the outermost layer that provides protection and pigmentation. The dermis is the middle layer that contains blood vessels, nerves, glands, hair follicles, and collagen. The hypodermis is the innermost layer that consists of fat and connective tissue.

The cells and molecules that make up your skin: Your skin is composed of different types of cells and molecules that perform various functions. The most common cells are keratinocytes, which produce keratin, a protein that gives your skin strength and elasticity. Other cells include melanocytes, which produce melanin, a pigment that gives your skin color and protects it from UV rays; Langerhans cells, which are part of your immune system and fight infections; and Merkel cells, which are sensory cells that detect touch and pressure. The most important molecules in your skin are collagen and elastin, which are fibrous proteins that provide structure and flexibility to your skin.

The blood vessels, nerves, and glands that nourish and regulate your skin: Your skin has a rich network of blood vessels, nerves, and glands that supply it with oxygen, nutrients, hormones, and signals. The blood vessels deliver blood to your skin and help regulate its temperature and healing. The nerves transmit sensations and impulses to and from your skin and brain. The glands secrete substances that lubricate, moisturize, and protect your skin. The most common glands are sebaceous glands, which produce sebum, an oily substance that prevents your skin from drying out; and sweat glands, which produce sweat, a watery substance that cools your skin and removes toxins.

The pigments, hairs, and nails that decorate and protect your skin: Your skin has various features that enhance and protect its appearance and function. The pigments are the colors that your skin produces or absorbs, such as melanin, carotene, and hemoglobin. The hairs are the thin strands that grow from your skin and serve as insulation, sensory receptors, and filters. The nails are the hard plates that cover the tips of your fingers and toes and provide support, protection, and grip.

The mechanisms of skin growth, repair, and renewal: Your skin is constantly growing, repairing, and renewing itself. The process of skin growth involves the division and differentiation of stem cells in the basal layer of the epidermis, which produce new keratinocytes that migrate to the surface and form the stratum corneum, the outermost layer of dead and flattened cells that shed off regularly. The process of skin repair involves the activation and migration of various cells, such as fibroblasts, macrophages, and platelets, that close and heal wounds, infections, and injuries. The process of skin renewal involves the turnover and replacement of old and damaged cells and molecules, such as collagen and elastin, that maintain the health and quality of your skin.

The factors that influence your skin health and appearance: Your skin health and appearance are influenced by many internal and external factors, such as genetics, age, hormones, diet, hydration, stress, sleep, smoking, alcohol, drugs, medications, sun exposure, pollution, climate, cosmetics, and skin care products. These factors can affect your skin positively or negatively, depending on their type, amount, frequency, and duration. Some factors can cause or worsen skin problems, such as acne, wrinkles, dryness, sensitivity, inflammation, infection, allergy, or cancer. Some factors can prevent or improve skin problems, such as antioxidants, vitamins, minerals, moisturizers, cleansers, exfoliators, toners, serums, masks, creams, sunscreens, and treatments.

The common skin disorders and diseases and how to prevent and treat them: Your skin can suffer from various disorders and diseases that affect its function and appearance. Some of the common skin disorders and diseases are: acne, which is a condition that occurs when your pores become clogged with oil, dirt, bacteria, and dead skin cells; eczema, which is a condition that causes your skin to become dry, itchy, red, and inflamed; psoriasis, which is a condition that causes your skin to produce too many cells that form thick, scaly, and red patches; rosacea, which is a condition that causes your skin to become red, swollen, and sensitive; dermatitis, which is a general term for any inflammation of the skin; fungal infections, which are infections caused by fungi that grow on your skin, such as ringworm, athlete's foot, and candidiasis; bacterial infections, which are infections caused by bacteria that invade your skin, such as impetigo, cellulitis, and staphylococcus; viral infections, which are infections caused by viruses that affect your skin, such as herpes, warts, and chickenpox; parasitic infections, which are infections caused by parasites that live on or in your skin, such as scabies, lice, and ticks; skin cancer, which is a condition that occurs when your skin cells grow abnormally and form tumors, such as basal cell carcinoma, squamous cell carcinoma, and melanoma. These skin disorders and diseases can be prevented and treated by various methods, such as hygiene, medication, therapy, surgery, or lifestyle changes.

The ways to measure and assess your skin condition and quality: Your skin condition and quality can be measured and assessed by various methods, such as observation, palpation, photography, imaging, testing, or analysis. These methods can help you determine your skin type, concerns, and goals, and evaluate your skin health and beauty. Some of the common methods are: observation, which is the visual inspection of your skin for its color, texture, tone, clarity, elasticity, firmness, smoothness, and radiance; palpation, which is the tactile examination of your skin for its temperature, moisture, oiliness, dryness, roughness, sensitivity, and pain; photography, which is the capture of your skin image by a camera or a smartphone for comparison, documentation, or diagnosis; imaging, which is the use of devices or techniques that produce images of your skin layers, structures, or functions, such as ultrasound, MRI, or thermography; testing, which is the use of instruments or kits that measure or detect certain aspects of your skin, such as pH, hydration, sebum, melanin, or elasticity; analysis, which is the use of software or algorithms that process or interpret your skin data, such as complexion analysis, skin age, or skin score.

The best practices and tips to maintain and improve your skin health and beauty: Your skin health and beauty can be maintained and improved by various practices and tips, such as skin care, nutrition, hydration, exercise, relaxation, sleep, protection, and enhancement. These practices and tips can help you keep your skin healthy, radiant, and beautiful. Some of the common practices and tips are: skin care, which is the routine of cleansing, toning, moisturizing, exfoliating, masking, treating, and protecting your skin with appropriate products and techniques; nutrition, which is the intake of foods and supplements that provide your skin with essential nutrients, such as antioxidants, vitamins, minerals, proteins, fats, and carbohydrates; hydration, which is the consumption of fluids and foods that provide your skin with water, such as water, juice, tea, fruits, and vegetables; exercise, which is the physical activity that improves your skin circulation, oxygenation, detoxification, and metabolism; relaxation, which is the mental activity that reduces your skin stress, tension, and inflammation; sleep, which is the restful state that repairs and rejuvenates your skin cells and molecules; protection, which is the prevention of your skin damage and aging by avoiding or minimizing exposure to harmful factors, such as sun, pollution, smoke, alcohol, drugs, or medications; enhancement, which is the improvement of your skin appearance and function by using or applying cosmetic or aesthetic products or procedures, such as makeup, hair removal, nail care, or botox.

Chapter 2

The different types of skin and how to identify your skin type

The different skin types and how to identify yours is a topic that explains the classification of skin based on its characteristics, such as oiliness, dryness, sensitivity, and reactivity. It also explains how to determine your own skin type by observing and testing your skin.

The five main skin types and their features: The five main skin types are normal, oily, dry, combination, and sensitive. Normal skin is balanced, smooth, and clear, with no excess oil or dryness. Oily skin is shiny, greasy, and prone to acne, blackheads, and enlarged pores. Dry skin is dull, flaky, and tight, with low moisture and elasticity. Combination skin is a mix of oily and dry areas, usually with an oily T-zone (forehead, nose, and chin) and dry cheeks. Sensitive skin is easily irritated, inflamed, and reddened, with reactions to various factors, such as products, ingredients, or environmental conditions.

The factors that affect your skin type: Your skin type is determined by various factors, such as genetics, hormones, age, climate, diet, hydration, stress, sleep, medication, and skin care products. These factors can change your skin type over time, or cause temporary or seasonal variations. For example, your skin may become more oily during puberty, pregnancy, or menstruation, due to hormonal changes. Your skin may become more dry during winter, due to cold and dry air. Your skin may become more sensitive due to allergies, infections, or injuries.

The methods to identify your skin type: There are several methods to identify your skin type, such as observation, touch, blotting, or testing. Observation is the simplest method, where you look at your skin in natural light and notice its appearance, texture, and condition. Touch is another method, where you feel your skin with your fingers and notice its temperature, moisture, oiliness, dryness, roughness, or smoothness. Blotting is a method where you use a tissue or a blotting paper to press on different areas of your face and notice the amount of oil or dirt that transfers onto the paper. Testing is a method where you use a device or a kit that measures certain aspects of your skin, such as pH, hydration, sebum, or elasticity.

Chapter 3

The factors that affect your skin health and appearance

The factors that affect your skin health and appearance is a topic that explains the various internal and external factors that influence how your skin looks and feels. It also explains how to prevent or minimize the negative effects of these factors, and how to enhance or maximize the positive effects of these factors.

The internal factors that affect your skin health and appearance: These are the factors that originate from within your body, such as genetics, hormones, age, diet, hydration, stress, sleep, medication, and illness. These factors can affect your skin positively or negatively, depending on their type, amount, frequency, and duration. For example, genetics can determine your skin type, color, and sensitivity, and make you more or less prone to certain skin problems, such as acne, eczema, or skin cancer. Hormones can regulate your skin oil production, collagen synthesis, and inflammation, and cause changes in your skin during puberty, pregnancy, or menopause. Age can affect your skin elasticity, firmness, and smoothness, and cause signs of aging, such as wrinkles, sagging, and spots. Diet can provide your skin with essential nutrients, such as antioxidants, vitamins, minerals, proteins, fats, and carbohydrates, and affect your skin health and beauty. Hydration can keep your skin moist, plump, and supple, and prevent your skin from drying out, cracking, or peeling. Stress can trigger your skin to produce more cortisol, a hormone that can increase your skin oiliness, breakouts, and inflammation, and impair your skin healing and immunity. Sleep can repair and rejuvenate your skin cells and molecules, and improve your skin circulation, oxygenation, and detoxification. Medication can affect your skin positively or negatively, depending on the drug, dose, and side effects. Illness can affect your skin health and appearance, depending on the disease, symptoms, and treatment.

The external factors that affect your skin health and appearance: These are the factors that originate from outside your body, such as sun exposure, pollution, climate, cosmetics, and skin care products. These factors can also affect your skin positively or negatively, depending on their type, amount, frequency, and duration. For example, sun exposure can provide your skin with vitamin D, a nutrient that helps your skin growth, repair, and immunity, and give your skin a healthy and natural glow. However, too much sun exposure can damage your skin cells and molecules, and cause sunburn, premature aging, and skin cancer. Pollution can expose your skin to harmful chemicals, particles, and gases, that can clog your pores, irritate your skin, and cause oxidative stress, inflammation, and infection. Climate can affect your skin moisture, temperature, and sensitivity, and cause your skin to adapt to different environmental conditions, such as heat, cold, humidity, or dryness. Cosmetics can enhance your skin appearance and function, by covering, correcting, or improving your skin features, such as color, texture, tone, or shape. However, some cosmetics can also harm your skin, by causing allergic reactions, irritation, or infection, or by containing toxic or harmful ingredients, such as parabens, sulfates, or phthalates. Skin care products can maintain and improve your skin health and beauty, by cleansing, toning, moisturizing, exfoliating, masking, treating, and protecting your skin with appropriate products and techniques. However, some skin care products can also damage your skin, by using the wrong products or techniques for your skin type, concerns, or goals, or by overusing or underusing certain products or techniques.

Chapter 4

The best skin care products, ingredients, and tools for your skin type and concerns

The best skin care products, ingredients, and tools for your skin type and concerns is a topic that explains the various types of products, ingredients, and tools that can help you achieve your skin care goals, depending on your skin type and concerns.

The types of skin care products and their functions: There are many types of skin care products that can perform different functions for your skin, such as cleansing, toning, moisturizing, exfoliating, masking, treating, and protecting. Cleansing products are used to remove dirt, oil, makeup, and impurities from your skin, such as cleansers, face washes, micellar waters, or makeup removers. Toning products are used to balance your skin pH, refine your pores, and prepare your skin for the next steps, such as toners, essences, or mists. Moisturizing products are used to hydrate, nourish, and soften your skin, such as moisturizers, creams, lotions, or oils. Exfoliating products are used to remove dead skin cells, unclog pores, and improve your skin texture and tone, such as scrubs, peels, or acids. Masking products are used to deliver concentrated ingredients, boost your skin benefits, and address specific concerns, such as masks, patches, or sheets. Treating products are used to target and correct your skin problems, such as acne, wrinkles, dark spots, or redness, such as serums, ampoules, or spot treatments. Protecting products are used to shield your skin from external factors, such as sun, pollution, or blue light, such as sunscreens, primers, or foundations.

The types of skin care ingredients and their benefits: There are many types of skin care ingredients that can provide different benefits for your skin, such as antioxidants, vitamins, minerals, proteins, fats, and carbohydrates. Antioxidants are ingredients that protect your skin from oxidative stress, inflammation, and aging, such as vitamin C, vitamin E, or green tea. Vitamins are ingredients that support your skin growth, repair, and immunity, such as vitamin A, vitamin B, or vitamin D. Minerals are ingredients that regulate your skin functions, such as zinc, magnesium, or copper. Proteins are ingredients that provide your skin with structure and flexibility, such as collagen, elastin, or keratin. Fats are ingredients that provide your skin with moisture and barrier, such as ceramides, fatty acids, or cholesterol. Carbohydrates are ingredients that provide your skin with energy and hydration, such as hyaluronic acid, glycerin, or glucose.

The types of skin care tools and their uses: There are many types of skin care tools that can enhance your skin care results, such as brushes, sponges, rollers, or devices. Brushes are tools that can help you apply, blend, or remove your skin care products, such as cleansing brushes, makeup brushes, or mask brushes. Sponges are tools that can help you absorb, distribute, or dab your skin care products, such as konjac sponges, beauty blenders, or cotton pads. Rollers are tools that can help you massage, stimulate, or cool your skin, such as jade rollers, ice rollers, or derma rollers. Devices are tools that can help you measure, analyze, or treat your skin, such as skin analyzers, LED lights, or microcurrents.

Chapter 5

The step-by-step skin care routine for morning and night

The step-by-step skin care routine for morning and night is a topic that explains the order and purpose of applying different skin care products and techniques in the morning and at night. It also explains how to customize your skin care routine according to your skin type and concerns.

The basic steps of a skin care routine: A skin care routine usually consists of four basic steps: cleansing, toning, moisturizing, and protecting. Cleansing is the first step that removes dirt, oil, makeup, and impurities from your skin, and prepares it for the next steps. Toning is the second step that balances your skin pH, refines your pores, and enhances the absorption of other products. Moisturizing is the third step that hydrates, nourishes, and softens your skin, and prevents it from drying out or cracking. Protecting is the fourth step that shields your skin from external factors, such as sun, pollution, or blue light, and prevents it from damage or aging.

The difference between a morning and a night skin care routine: A morning and a night skin care routine have some similarities and differences. The similarities are that they both follow the basic steps of cleansing, toning, moisturizing, and protecting, and they both use products and techniques that suit your skin type and concerns. The differences are that a morning skin care routine focuses more on protecting your skin from the day ahead, while a night skin care routine focuses more on repairing your skin from the day behind. A morning skin care routine usually uses lighter and simpler products, such as a gentle cleanser, a hydrating toner, a lightweight moisturizer, and a broad-spectrum sunscreen. A night skin care routine usually uses heavier and more complex products, such as a double cleanser, an exfoliating toner, a rich moisturizer, and a treatment product.

The additional steps of a skin care routine: A skin care routine can also include some additional steps that can boost your skin benefits and address specific concerns, such as exfoliating, masking, treating, and enhancing. Exfoliating is a step that removes dead skin cells, unclogs pores, and improves your skin texture and tone, and can be done once or twice a week, depending on your skin type and sensitivity. Masking is a step that delivers concentrated ingredients, boosts your skin benefits, and addresses specific concerns, and can be done once or twice a week, or as needed, depending on your skin type and needs. Treating is a step that targets and corrects your skin problems, such as acne, wrinkles, dark spots, or redness, and can be done daily or as needed, depending on your skin type and goals. Enhancing is a step that improves your skin appearance and function, by using or applying cosmetic or aesthetic products or procedures, such as makeup, hair removal, nail care, or botox, and can be done daily or occasionally, depending on your personal preferences and occasions.

The examples of a skin care routine for different skin types and concerns: A skin care routine can be customized according to your skin type and concerns, by choosing the right products, ingredients, and techniques for your skin. Here are some examples of a skin care routine for different skin types and concerns:

Normal skin: Normal skin is balanced, smooth, and clear, with no excess oil or dryness. A skin care routine for normal skin can be simple and basic, using products and ingredients that maintain and enhance your skin health and beauty. For example, a morning skin care routine for normal skin can consist of: a gentle cleanser, a hydrating toner, a lightweight moisturizer, and a broad-spectrum sunscreen. A night skin care routine for normal skin can consist of: a gentle cleanser, a hydrating toner, a rich moisturizer, and a treatment product, such as a serum, an ampoule, or a spot treatment, that targets your specific concern or goal, such as anti-aging, brightening, or soothing.

Oily skin: Oily skin is shiny, greasy, and prone to acne, blackheads, and enlarged pores. A skin care routine for oily skin can be focused on controlling your oil production, clearing your pores, and preventing your breakouts. For example, a morning skin care routine for oily skin can consist of: a foaming cleanser, a clarifying toner, a gel moisturizer, and a mattifying sunscreen. A night skin care routine for oily skin can consist of: a double cleanser, an exfoliating toner, a gel moisturizer, and a treatment product, such as a serum, an ampoule, or a spot treatment, that contains ingredients that regulate your oil, such as salicylic acid, niacinamide, or tea tree oil.

Dry skin: Dry skin is dull, flaky, and tight, with low moisture and elasticity. A skin care routine for dry skin can be focused on restoring your moisture, nourishing your skin, and improving your skin barrier. For example, a morning skin care routine for dry skin can consist of: a cream cleanser, a moisturizing toner, a cream moisturizer, and a hydrating sunscreen. A night skin care routine for dry skin can consist of: a cream cleanser, a moisturizing toner, a cream moisturizer, and a treatment product, such as a serum, an ampoule, or a spot treatment, that contains ingredients that hydrate your skin, such as hyaluronic acid, glycerin, or ceramides.

Combination skin: Combination skin is a mix of oily and dry areas, usually with an oily T-zone (forehead, nose, and chin) and dry cheeks. A skin care routine for combination skin can be focused on balancing your oil and moisture, and addressing your different concerns. For example, a morning skin care routine for combination skin can consist of: a gel cleanser, a balancing toner, a lotion moisturizer, and a lightweight sunscreen. A night skin care routine for combination skin can consist of: a gel cleanser, a balancing toner, a lotion moisturizer, and a treatment product, such as a serum, an ampoule, or a spot treatment, that targets your specific concern or goal, such as anti-aging, brightening, or soothing, and can be applied to different areas of your face, depending on your needs.

Sensitive skin: Sensitive skin is easily irritated, inflamed, and reddened, with reactions to various factors, such as products, ingredients, or environmental conditions. A skin care routine for sensitive skin can be focused on calming your skin, reducing your inflammation, and avoiding your triggers. For example, a morning skin care routine for sensitive skin can consist of: a gentle cleanser, a soothing toner, a gentle moisturizer, and a mineral sunscreen. A night skin care routine for sensitive skin can consist of: a gentle cleanser, a soothing toner, a gentle moisturizer, and a treatment product, such as a serum, an ampoule, or a spot treatment, that contains ingredients that soothe your skin, such as aloe vera, chamomile, or oatmeal.

Chapter 6

The "dos" and "don'ts" of skin care

The dos and don'ts of skin care is a topic that explains the best practices and the common mistakes of skin care, and how to avoid or correct them. You will learn:

The "dos" of skin care

These are the things that you should do to keep your skin healthy, radiant, and beautiful. Some of the dos of skin care are:

Do know your skin type and concerns, and choose the right products, ingredients, and techniques for your skin.

Do follow a consistent and regular skin care routine, both in the morning and at night, and adjust it according to your skin needs and changes.

Do cleanse your skin gently and thoroughly, using lukewarm water and a gentle cleanser, and pat it dry with a soft towel.

Do tone your skin after cleansing, using a toner that suits your skin type and concerns, and apply it with a cotton pad or your fingers.

Do moisturize your skin after toning, using a moisturizer that suits your skin type and concerns, and apply it with your fingers or a brush.

Do exfoliate your skin once or twice a week, using a scrub, a peel, or an acid, and apply it with your fingers or a brush, and rinse it off with water.

Do mask your skin once or twice a week, or as needed, using a mask that suits your skin type and concerns, and apply it with your fingers or a brush, and leave it on for the recommended time, and rinse it off with water or tissue it off.

Do treat your skin problems, such as acne, wrinkles, dark spots, or redness, using a treatment product, such as a serum, an ampoule, or a spot treatment, and apply it with your fingers or a dropper, and target the affected areas or the whole face.

Do protect your skin from external factors, such as sun, pollution, or blue light, using a protection product, such as a sunscreen, a primer, or a foundation, and apply it with your fingers or a sponge, and cover the exposed areas or the whole face.

Do enhance your skin appearance and function, using cosmetic or aesthetic products or procedures, such as makeup, hair removal, nail care, or botox, and apply or perform them with the appropriate tools or techniques, and follow the instructions or recommendations.

Do nourish your skin from within, by eating a balanced and healthy diet, drinking enough water, taking supplements, and avoiding smoking, alcohol, or drugs.

Do exercise your skin, by doing physical activities that improve your skin circulation, oxygenation, detoxification, and metabolism, and by doing facial exercises that tone your facial muscles and prevent sagging.

Do relax your skin, by reducing your stress levels, practicing meditation, yoga, or breathing exercises, and by using aromatherapy, massage, or acupressure.

Do sleep your skin, by getting enough and quality sleep, following a good sleep hygiene, and by using silk pillowcases, eye masks, or humidifiers.

Do measure and assess your skin condition and quality, by using devices or kits that measure or detect certain aspects of your skin, such as pH, hydration, sebum, or elasticity, and by using software or algorithms that process or interpret your skin data, such as complexion analysis, skin age, or skin score.

The don'ts of skin care

These are the things that you should avoid or minimize to prevent your skin damage, aging, and problems. Some of the don'ts of skin care are:

Don't use the wrong products or techniques for your skin type, concerns, or goals, as they can cause irritation, inflammation, or infection, or worsen your skin condition or appearance.

Don't skip or neglect any steps of your skin care routine, as they can compromise your skin health and beauty, or reduce the effectiveness of other products or techniques.

Don't overuse or underuse any products or techniques, as they can either dry out, strip, or sensitize your skin, or leave behind residues, clogs, or impurities on your skin.

Don't use expired or contaminated products, as they can lose their potency, quality, or safety, or harbor harmful bacteria, fungi, or toxins that can infect or poison your skin.

Don't share your products or tools with others, as they can transfer germs, dirt, or oil from one person to another, and cause cross-contamination or infection.

Don't touch, pick, or pop your skin, especially your pimples, blackheads, or scabs, as they can introduce bacteria, dirt, or oil into your skin, and cause inflammation, infection, or scarring.

Don't expose your skin to excessive or harmful factors, such as sun, pollution, or blue light, as they can damage your skin cells and molecules, and cause sunburn, premature aging, or skin cancer.

Don't use harsh or abrasive products or tools, such as alcohol, sulfates, or scrubs, as they can strip your skin of its natural oils and moisture, and cause dryness, irritation, or sensitivity.

Don't use products or ingredients that you are allergic or sensitive to, as they can trigger your skin to react with redness, swelling, itching, or rash, and cause discomfort or pain.

Don't use products or ingredients that are toxic or harmful, such as parabens, phthalates, or mercury, as they can accumulate in your body and cause adverse effects, such as hormonal disruption, organ damage, or cancer.

Don't eat or drink unhealthy or unbalanced foods or fluids, such as junk food, sugar, caffeine, or alcohol, as they can deprive your skin of essential nutrients, and cause inflammation, dehydration, or breakouts.

Don't exercise too much or too little, as they can either stress out, exhaust, or overheat your skin, or make your skin sluggish, dull, or saggy.

Don't relax too much or too little, as they can either make your skin lazy, bored, or depressed, or make your skin tense, anxious, or angry.

Don't sleep too much or too little, as they can either make your skin puffy, pale, or oily, or make your skin dark, wrinkled, or dry

Chapter 7

The common skin care myths and misconceptions

The common skin care myths and misconceptions is a topic that explains the false or misleading beliefs or ideas about skin care, and how to correct or debunk them. You will learn:

The common skin care myths and misconceptions and their sources

There are many common skin care myths and misconceptions that are spread by various sources, such as media, marketing, celebrities, or word-of-mouth. Some of these misconceptions and myths are:

Myth: The more expensive a product is, the better it is for your skin.

Source: Marketing, media, or celebrities that promote or endorse high-end or luxury products, and create a perception of quality, effectiveness, or status.

Myth: The more products or ingredients you use, the better it is for your skin.

Source: Media, marketing, or word-of-mouth that suggest or recommend multiple or complex products or ingredients, and create a perception of necessity, variety, or completeness.

Myth: The more natural or organic a product is, the better it is for your skin.

Source: Media, marketing, or celebrities that promote or endorse natural or organic products, and create a perception of safety, purity, or sustainability.

Myth: You don't need sunscreen if it's cloudy, rainy, or winter.

Source: Media, marketing, or word-of-mouth that suggest or recommend sunscreen only for sunny, hot, or summer days, and create a perception of protection, comfort, or convenience.

Myth: You don't need moisturizer if you have oily skin.

Source: Media, marketing, or word-of-mouth that suggest or recommend moisturiser only for dry skin,

and create a perception of oiliness, greasiness, or breakouts.

Myth: You can use the same products or techniques for your face and body.

Source: Media, marketing, or word-of-mouth that suggest or recommend products or techniques that are suitable for both face and body, and create a perception of simplicity, efficiency, or economy.

The common skin care myths and misconceptions and their truths

There are many common skin care myths and misconceptions that are contradicted or refuted by scientific evidence, expert opinion, or personal experience. Some of these myths and misconceptions and their truths are:

Myth: The more expensive a product is, the better it is for your skin.

Truth: The price of a product does not necessarily reflect its quality, effectiveness, or suitability for your skin. A product's price is influenced by many factors, such as brand, packaging, marketing, or distribution, that may not have anything to do with its performance or benefits for your skin. A product's quality, effectiveness, or suitability for your skin depends on its ingredients, formulation, concentration, stability, and compatibility with your skin type and concerns. You can find good or bad products in any price range, and you should choose a product based on its ingredients, formulation, concentration, stability, and compatibility with your skin type and concerns, not its price.

Myth: The more products or ingredients you use, the better it is for your skin.

Truth: The number of products or ingredients you use does not necessarily reflect their necessity, variety, or completeness for your skin. A product's number is influenced by many factors, such as marketing, trends, or preferences, that may not have anything to do with its function or benefits for your skin. A product's necessity, variety, or completeness for your skin depends on its function, benefits, and synergy with other products or ingredients. You can use too many or too few products or ingredients for your skin, and you should use a product based on its function, benefits, and synergy with other products or ingredients, not its number.

Myth: The more natural or organic a product is, the better it is for your skin.

Truth: The origin of a product does not necessarily reflect its safety, purity, or sustainability for your skin. A product's origin is influenced by many factors, such as regulation, certification, or definition, that may not have anything to do with its safety, purity, or sustainability for your skin. A product's safety, purity, or sustainability for your skin depends on its ingredients, formulation, concentration, stability, and compatibility with your skin type and concerns. You can find safe or unsafe, pure or impure, sustainable or unsustainable products in any origin, and you should choose a product based on its ingredients, formulation, concentration, stability, and compatibility with your skin type and concerns, not its origin.

Myth: You don't need sunscreen if it's cloudy, rainy, or winter.

Truth: The weather or season does not necessarily reflect the intensity or duration of the sun's rays for your skin. The sun's rays are influenced by many factors, such as latitude, altitude, time, or reflection, that may not have anything to do with the weather or season. The sun's rays can damage your skin cells and molecules, and cause sunburn, premature aging, or skin cancer, regardless of the weather or season. You need sunscreen every day, all year round, and you should apply a sunscreen that has a broad-spectrum protection, a high SPF, and a water-resistant formula, and reapply it every two hours or after sweating or swimming, not based on the weather or season.

Myth: You don't need moisturiser if you have oily skin.

Truth: The oiliness or dryness of your skin does not necessarily reflect the hydration or nourishment of your skin. The oiliness or dryness of your skin is influenced by many factors, such as genetics, hormones, age, or climate, that may not have anything to do with the hydration or nourishment of your skin. The hydration or nourishment of your skin depends on its water and oil content, and its ability to retain them.

You need moisturizer regardless of your skin type, and you should use a moisturizer that suits your skin type and concerns, and apply it after cleansing and toning, not based on the oiliness or dryness of your skin.

Myth: You can use the same products or techniques for your face and body.

Truth: The face and body of your skin do not necessarily have the same characteristics, needs, or preferences. The face and body of your skin are influenced by many factors, such as exposure, sensitivity, or function, that may not have anything to do with each other. The face and body of your skin may have different skin types, concerns, or goals, and may require different products, ingredients, or techniques. You should use different products or techniques for your face and body, and choose them based on their suitability for each part, not based on their similarity or difference.

Chapter 8

The tips and tricks to enhance your skin care results

The tips and tricks to enhance your skin care results is a topic that explains the various ways to improve your skin health and beauty, by using or applying some simple or creative methods or techniques.

The tips and tricks to enhance your skin care results and their sources: There are many tips and tricks to enhance your skin care results that are derived from various sources, such as science, tradition, culture, or innovation. Some of these tips and tricks are:

Tip: Use a cold spoon or ice cube to depuff your eyes in the morning.

Source: Science, as cold temperature can constrict your blood vessels and reduce swelling and inflammation.

Tip: Use honey as a natural moisturizer, antibacterial, or anti-inflammatory agent for your skin.

Source: Tradition, as honey has been used for centuries as a remedy for various skin conditions, such as dryness, acne, or wounds.

Tip: Use rice water as a toner, cleanser, or mask for your skin.

Source: Culture, as rice water is a popular ingredient in Asian beauty rituals, as it contains vitamins, minerals, and antioxidants that can brighten, soften, and nourish your skin.

Tip: Use a jade roller or a gua sha tool to massage, stimulate, or sculpt your face.

Source: Innovation, as these are modern tools that are inspired by ancient Chinese practices, as they can improve your skin circulation, oxygenation, detoxification, and metabolism, and tone your facial muscles and prevent sagging.

The tips and tricks to enhance your skin care results and their benefits: There are many tips and tricks to enhance your skin care results that can provide different benefits for your skin, such as hydration, nourishment, protection, correction, or enhancement. Some of these tips and tricks and their benefits are:

Tip: Use a cold spoon or ice cube to depuff your eyes in the morning.

Benefit: This tip can help you reduce the appearance of eye bags, dark circles, or puffiness, and make your eyes look more awake, alert, and refreshed.

Tip: Use honey as a natural moisturizer, antibacterial, or anti-inflammatory agent for your skin.

Benefit: This tip can help you hydrate, heal, and soothe your skin, and prevent or treat various skin problems, such as dryness, acne, or inflammation.

Tip: Use rice water as a toner, cleanser, or mask for your skin.

Benefit: This tip can help you cleanse, tone, and moisturize your skin, and improve your skin texture, tone, and clarity.

Tip: Use a jade roller or a gua sha tool to massage, stimulate, or sculpt your face.

Benefit: This tip can help you relax, rejuvenate, and beautify your face, and enhance your skin health and appearance.

Chapter 9

The natural and DIY skin care alternatives

The natural and DIY skin care alternatives is a topic that explains the various ways to use natural or homemade products or ingredients for your skin care, instead of or in addition to commercial or synthetic products or ingredients.

The reasons to use natural and DIY skin care alternatives: There are many reasons to use natural and DIY skin care alternatives, such as:

To save money, as natural and DIY skin care alternatives are usually cheaper and more accessible than commercial or synthetic products or ingredients.

To avoid chemicals, as natural and DIY skin care alternatives are usually free of or low in artificial or harmful chemicals, such as parabens, sulfates, or phthalates, that can cause adverse effects on your skin or health.

To customize your skin care, as natural and DIY skin care alternatives are usually more flexible and adaptable than commercial or synthetic products or ingredients, and you can adjust them according to your skin type, concerns, or preferences.

To have fun, as natural and DIY skin care alternatives are usually more creative and enjoyable than commercial or synthetic products or ingredients, and you can experiment with different recipes, methods, or techniques.

The types of natural and DIY skin care alternatives and their functions: There are many types of natural and DIY skin care alternatives that can perform different functions for your skin, such as cleansing, toning, moisturizing, exfoliating, masking, treating, and protecting. Some of the types of natural and DIY skin care alternatives are:

Oils, such as olive oil, coconut oil, or jojoba oil, that can be used to cleanse, moisturize, or protect your skin, as they can dissolve dirt, oil, and makeup, and provide your skin with moisture and barrier.

Vinegars, such as apple cider vinegar or white vinegar, that can be used to tone or treat your skin, as they can balance your skin pH, refine your pores, and fight bacteria and fungi.

Fruits, such as lemon, banana, or avocado, that can be used to moisturize, exfoliate, or mask your skin, as they can provide your skin with water, vitamins, minerals, and antioxidants, and remove dead skin cells and brighten your skin tone.

 Vegetables, such as cucumber, potato, or tomato, that can be used to moisturize, soothe, or treat your skin, as they can provide your skin with water, vitamins, minerals, and antioxidants, and reduce inflammation, redness, or dark spots.

Herbs, such as aloe vera, chamomile, or lavender, that can be used to moisturize, soothe, or treat your skin, as they can provide your skin with water, vitamins, minerals, and antioxidants, and reduce inflammation, irritation, or infection.

Spices, such as turmeric, cinnamon, or ginger, that can be used to exfoliate, mask, or treat your skin, as they can provide your skin with vitamins, minerals, and antioxidants, and stimulate your skin circulation, oxygenation, and detoxification, and fight bacteria and fungi.

Sugars, such as brown sugar, white sugar, or honey, that can be used to exfoliate, moisturize, or treat your skin, as they can provide your skin with carbohydrates, and remove dead skin cells and improve your skin texture and tone, and hydrate, heal, and soothe your skin.

Salts, such as sea salt, Himalayan salt, or Epsom salt, that can be used to exfoliate, cleanse, or treat your skin, as they can provide your skin with minerals, and remove dead skin cells and improve your skin texture and tone, and draw out impurities and toxins from your skin.

Milks, such as cow milk, goat milk, or almond milk, that can be used to cleanse, moisturize, or mask your skin, as they can provide your skin with proteins, fats, and carbohydrates, and dissolve dirt, oil, and makeup, and hydrate, nourish, and soften your skin.

 Yoghourts, such as plain yogurt, Greek yogurt, or probiotic yogurt, that can be used to cleanse, moisturize, or mask your skin, as they can provide your skin with proteins, fats, and carbohydrates, and dissolve dirt, oil, and makeup, and hydrate, nourish, and soften your skin, and balance your skin flora and fight bacteria and fungi.

 Eggs, such as whole eggs, egg whites, or egg yolks, that can be used to moisturize, tighten, or mask your skin, as they can provide your skin with proteins, fats, and vitamins, and hydrate, nourish, and soften your skin, and firm, lift, and smooth your skin.

Teas, such as green tea, black tea, or chamomile tea, that can be used to tone, soothe, or treat your skin, as they can provide your skin with water, vitamins, minerals, and antioxidants, and balance your skin pH, refine your pores, and reduce inflammation, irritation, or infection.

Clays, such as bentonite clay, kaolin clay, or French green clay, that can be used to cleanse, exfoliate, or mask your skin, as they can provide your skin with minerals, and draw out impurities, toxins, and excess oil from your skin, and improve your skin texture and tone.

Oatmeals, such as rolled oats, steel-cut oats, or oat flour, that can be used to cleanse, exfoliate, or mask your skin, as they can provide your skin with carbohydrates, proteins, and fats, and dissolve dirt, oil, and makeup, and remove dead skin cells and improve your skin texture and tone, and hydrate, nourish, and soothe your skin.

Chapter 10

The skin care recommendations for different ages, seasons, and occasions

The skin care recommendations for different ages, seasons, and occasions is a topic that explains the various ways to adapt your skin care routine according to your age, season, or occasion, and how to achieve your skin care goals in different situations.

The skin care recommendations for different ages and their reasons: There are different skin care recommendations for different ages, as your skin changes over time, and requires different products, ingredients, and techniques to suit your skin type, concerns, and goals. Some of the skin care recommendations for different ages are:

Teens: Teens have skin that is usually oily, acne-prone, and sensitive, due to hormonal changes, stress, or lifestyle factors. A skin care routine for teens should be focused on controlling oil production, clearing pores, and preventing breakouts. Some of the skin care recommendations for teens are:

Use a gentle foaming cleanser twice a day, to remove dirt, oil, and makeup, and prevent clogged pores and acne.

Use a clarifying toner after cleansing, to balance your skin pH, refine your pores, and remove any residue.

Use a lightweight gel moisturizer after toning, to hydrate your skin without making it greasy or shiny.

Use a treatment product, such as a serum, an ampoule, or a spot treatment, that contains ingredients that regulate oil and fight bacteria, such as salicylic acid, niacinamide, or tea tree oil, and apply it to the affected areas or the whole face, as needed.

Use a broad-spectrum sunscreen every day, to protect your skin from sun damage and premature aging, and choose a formula that is oil-free, non-comedogenic, and mattifying.

Exfoliate your skin once or twice a week, using a gentle scrub, peel, or acid, to remove dead skin cells, unclog pores, and improve your skin texture and tone.

Mask your skin once or twice a week, or as needed, using a clay, charcoal, or mud mask, to draw out impurities, toxins, and excess oil from your skin, and improve your skin clarity and brightness.

Twenties: Twenties have skin that is usually normal, combination, or dry, depending on their genetics, hormones, or environment. A skin care routine for twenties should be focused on maintaining and enhancing your skin health and beauty, and preventing or delaying the signs of aging. Some of the skin care recommendations for twenties are:

- Use a gentle cream cleanser twice a day, to remove dirt, oil, and makeup, and nourish your skin.

- Use a hydrating toner after cleansing, to balance your skin pH, refine your pores, and enhance the absorption of other products.

- Use a lotion moisturizer after toning, to hydrate, nourish, and soften your skin, and prevent it from drying out or cracking.

- Use a treatment product, such as a serum, an ampoule, or a spot treatment, that contains ingredients that target your specific concern or goal, such as anti-aging, brightening, or soothing, and apply it to the affected areas or the whole face, as needed.

- Use a broad-spectrum sunscreen every day, to protect your skin from sun damage and premature aging, and choose a formula that is lightweight, non-greasy, and moisturizing.

- Exfoliate your skin once or twice a week, using a gentle scrub, peel, or acid, to remove dead skin cells, unclog pores, and improve your skin texture and tone.

- Mask your skin once or twice a week, or as needed, using a sheet, gel, or cream mask, to deliver concentrated ingredients, boost your skin benefits, and address specific concerns.

Thirties: Thirties have skin that is usually normal, dry, or sensitive, depending on their genetics, hormones, or environment. A skin care routine for thirties should be focused on restoring and improving your skin health and beauty, and treating or correcting the signs of aging. Some of the skin care recommendations for thirties are:

- Use a gentle cream cleanser twice a day, to remove dirt, oil, and makeup, and nourish your skin.

- Use an exfoliating toner after cleansing, to balance your skin pH, refine your pores, and remove any residue, and improve your skin texture and tone.

- Use a rich moisturizer after toning, to hydrate, nourish, and soften your skin, and prevent it from drying out or cracking.

- Use a treatment product, such as a serum, an ampoule, or a spot treatment, that contains ingredients that target your specific concern or goal, such as anti-aging, brightening, or soothing, and apply it to the affected areas or the whole face, as needed.

- Use a broad-spectrum sunscreen every day, to protect your skin from sun damage and premature aging, and choose a formula that is rich, creamy, and hydrating.

- Exfoliate your skin once or twice a week, using a gentle scrub, peel, or acid, to remove dead skin cells, unclog pores, and improve your skin texture and tone.

- Mask your skin once or twice a week, or as needed, using a sheet, gel, or cream mask, to deliver concentrated ingredients, boost your skin benefits, and address specific concerns.

Forties and beyond: Forties and beyond have skin that is usually dry, sensitive, or mature, depending on their genetics, hormones, or environment. A skin care routine for forties and beyond should be focused on repairing and rejuvenating your skin health and beauty, and reversing or minimizing the signs of aging. Some of the skin care recommendations for forties and beyond are:

- Use a gentle cream cleanser twice a day, to remove dirt, oil, and makeup, and nourish your skin.

- Use an exfoliating toner after cleansing, to balance your skin pH, refine your pores, and remove any residue, and improve your skin texture and tone.

- Use a rich moisturizer after toning, to hydrate, nourish, and soften your skin, and prevent it from drying out or cracking.

- Use a treatment product, such as a serum, an ampoule, or a spot treatment, that contains ingredients that target your specific concern or goal, such as anti-aging, brightening, or soothing, and apply it to the affected areas or the whole face, as needed.

- Use a broad-spectrum sunscreen every day, to protect your skin from sun damage and premature aging, and choose a formula that is rich, creamy, and hydrating.

- Exfoliate your skin once or twice a week, using a gentle scrub, peel, or acid, to remove dead skin cells, unclog pores, and improve your skin texture and tone.

- Mask your skin once or twice a week, or as needed, using a sheet, gel, or cream mask, to deliver concentrated ingredients, boost your skin benefits, and address specific concerns.

The skin care recommendations for different seasons and their reasons: There are different skin care recommendations for different seasons, as your skin changes with the weather, and requires different products, ingredients, and techniques to suit your skin type, concerns, and goals. Some of the skin care recommendations for different seasons are:

Spring: Spring is a season of transition, where your skin adapts from the cold and dry winter to the warm and humid summer. A skin care routine for spring should be focused on refreshing and renewing your skin, and preparing it for the summer ahead. Some of the skin care recommendations for spring are:

Use a gentle foaming cleanser twice a day, to remove dirt, oil, and makeup, and prevent clogged pores and acne.

Use a hydrating toner after cleansing, to balance your skin pH, refine your pores, and enhance the absorption of other products.

Use a lightweight lotion moisturizer after toning, to hydrate, nourish, and soften your skin, and prevent it from drying out or cracking.

Use a treatment product, such as a serum, an ampoule, or a spot treatment, that contains ingredients that target your specific concern or goal, such as anti-aging, brightening, or soothing, and apply it to the affected areas or the whole face, as needed.

Use a broad-spectrum sunscreen every day, to protect your skin from sun damage and premature aging, and choose a formula that is lightweight, non-greasy, and moisturizing.

 Exfoliate your skin once or twice a week, using a gentle scrub, peel, or acid, to remove dead skin cells, unclog pores, and improve your skin texture and tone, and reveal your fresh and radiant skin.

 Mask your skin once or twice a week, or as needed, using a sheet, gel, or cream mask, to deliver concentrated ingredients, boost your skin benefits, and address specific concerns, and hydrate, nourish, and brighten your skin.

 Summer: Summer is a season of heat, humidity, and sun, where your skin is exposed to high temperatures, sweat, and UV rays. A skin care routine for summer should be focused on cooling and protecting your skin, and preventing or treating sunburn, breakouts, or pigmentation. Some of the skin care recommendations for summer are:

Use a gentle foaming cleanser twice a day, to remove dirt, oil, and makeup, and prevent clogged pores and acne.

Use a clarifying toner after cleansing, to balance your skin pH, refine your pores, and remove any residue.

 Use a gel moisturizer after toning, to hydrate your skin without making it greasy or shiny.

Chapter 11

The skin care secrets of celebrities and experts

The skin care secrets of celebrities and experts is a topic that explains the various tips, tricks, and routines that celebrities and experts use or recommend to achieve and maintain healthy and beautiful skin.

The importance of hydration, sleep, and diet for skin health and beauty: Many celebrities and experts emphasize the role of hydration, sleep, and diet in keeping their skin radiant, smooth, and clear. For example, Lea Michele says that drinking a lot of water and getting a lot of sleep are the most important factors for her skin. Olivia Culpo says that eating more greens and avoiding processed foods help her skin glow. Gwyneth Paltrow is one of the most active supporters of drinking water, and she also advocates for a balanced and healthy diet that includes antioxidants, vitamins, minerals, proteins, fats, and carbohydrates.

The benefits of exfoliation, masking, and treatment for skin texture, tone, and clarity: Many celebrities and experts use or recommend exfoliation, masking, and treatment products or techniques to improve their skin texture, tone, and clarity. For example, Christie Brinkley says that she exfoliates her face every day, as she believes that it helps her skin feel fresh and smooth. Padma Lakshmi says that she uses honey as a natural moisturizer, antibacterial, and anti-inflammatory agent for her skin. Rihanna says that she uses a sheet mask before every red carpet event, as it helps her skin look plump and hydrated.

The advantages of natural and DIY skin care alternatives for skin safety, purity, and sustainability: Many celebrities and experts use or prefer natural and DIY skin care alternatives, as they are free of or low in artificial or harmful chemicals, and they can be customized according to their skin type, concerns, or preferences. For example, Cate Blanchett says that she uses olive oil and macadamia oil to cleanse and moisturize her skin. Gracie Abrams says that she uses ice cubes to depuff and cool her skin. Jennifer Lopez says that she uses a homemade mask made of oatmeal, yogurt, and honey to nourish and soothe her skin.

The use of tools and devices to enhance and optimize skin care results: Many celebrities and experts use or suggest tools and devices that can enhance and optimize their skin care results, such as brushes, sponges, rollers, or devices. For example, Kylie Jenner says that she uses a cleansing brush to remove dirt, oil, and makeup from her skin. Cindy Crawford says that she uses a jade roller to massage, stimulate, and sculpt her face. Jessica Alba says that she uses a LED light therapy device to keep her acne at bay.

Skin Care and You is more than just a book. It is a personal skin care coach that will help you achieve your skin care goals and transform your skin for the better. By following the advice and tips in this book, you will not only improve your skin condition and appearance, but also boost your self-esteem and confidence. You will feel good in your own skin, and enjoy the benefits of having a healthy and glowing complexion.